NATURAL

CURES

FOR

DEPRESSION

Dedicated To My Loving Family And
My Blessed Children

In the early eighties about three and a half years into a domestic violence marriage to the father of my children is when I began marriage counseling.

It wasn't long after that when I learned I had developed "*Situation Depression*" as a result of the **abuse** which later caused a divorce and severe financial hardship.

The *marriage counselor* had clued me in to the fact that I was married to an *abuser*. And she figured out that he wasn't willing to change.

Then she convinced me that I needed to think about me and my children as my priority.

She started helping me find a way to escape that grip he had me in for so many years.

It wasn't until decades later before I would realize the damage he had done to my self esteem that would last for over twenty years after I had escaped his grip.

The marriage counselor tried some different *anti depressants* on me but I really felt no change or difference at all.

Years went by and I moved out of state but I continued seeing a counselor so that I could try different anti depressants.

We tried so many of them all together maybe 25 or more. None of them ever worked.

Two of them actually made me feel really strange like I was dead to emotions so I had to stop that one quickly.

Finally, the counselor confirmed what all the other counselors had already told me that made me feel totally helpless.

They said I had "*Situational Depression*" and that nothing would help very much at all until the situation changed.

Since my situation was financial because I didn't have enough money to take care of my kids or enough resources to take care of them and with my severe back pain from previous injuries it only made it worse.

I didn't really feel depressed so to speak I just felt helpless and like a victim to circumstances.

Even worse was when my doctor was looking at all my prescriptions after I had been in a car accident in 1991 and he said "*What are you doing taking this?*" (He named my anti depressant) and I told him why I took it and he said "*you really shouldn't be taking that because it is making your* **congestive heart failure** *worse*" and I said "*What congestive heart failure*" and he said "*You have Edema Level Two Congestive heart failure.*"

As it turned out one of the arthritis medicines that my doctor had put me on was causing people to develop serious heart conditions.

That was just another anti depressant that they tried me on but didn't do one thing for me other than take up space in my digestive system and medicine cabinet.

They have since removed the arthritis medicine that caused people serious heart conditions from off of the market now.

Many years later (over twenty) I finally really did get the real feeling of depression. It only happened after about 2008 while I had returned to Missouri for the first time since I was a child.

I remember the first winter there I became really gloomy. They had called it the "*Winter blues*" and it is true that people really do get them.

The problem is a shortage of mainly *Vitamin D* but also they should take *Selenium* to help with light absorption.

But neither Vitamin D or Selenium were strong enough to fight the feeling of darkness that I only felt occasionally while living in **Missouri** throughout different times of the year even if the sun had been shining for days.

First of all, I learned that it needed to be addressed from a spiritual point of view as I was taught by some Christians who prayed for me on other occasions.

I knew that God had given me power to bind and to loose and that everything in heaven and earth has to submit to the name and authority of Christ Jesus.

I also knew that Jesus was a healer and that HE has already provided complete physical, mental and emotional healing from *Isaiah chapter fifty eight* "**By HIS stripes we are healed**"

So for the first time I began to take spiritual authority over that feeling while in Missouri. And I would pray like this : "*I bind every spirit of depression and darkness and I command you to take your hands off of me and off of my life. Leave now In the name of Jesus!*" And to my shock and surprise it would dissipate.

But I only started doing that after I had already learned about amino acids, brain salts and proteins that are naturally occurring in the brain from Dr. Eric Braverman of Path Medical in New York.

Dr. Eric R. Braverman MD

304 Park Ave
New York, NY
(212) 213-6155

www.pathmed.com

Take his *free* Brain Quiz here

And take his *free* Age Print Test here

Find all of them here on this page

I am so thankful for Dr. Braverman for sharing this wonderful medical information with me as it cured me of a 25 year long battle with *Situational Depression* as soon as I implemented Dr. Braverman's recommendations which I will share with you in this book.

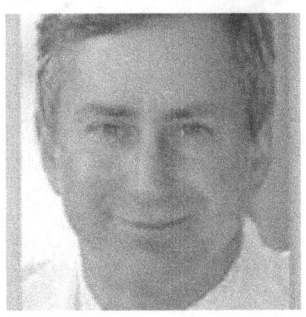

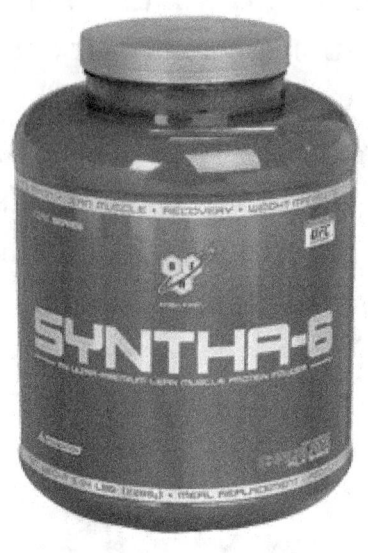

I learned about how brain <u>proteins</u>, natural brain salts and amino acids can counter set mid life hormone imbalances for men and women.

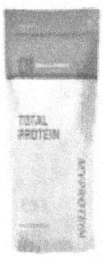

And that men also go through a period of a type of "*man-opause*" but its medical term is ***Andropause***.

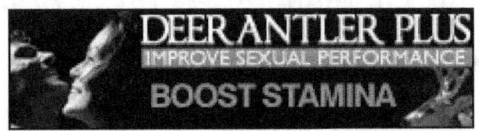

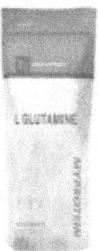

Men and women both can sometimes be treated from these mid life hormonal imbalances with simple supplements of these *brain salts, amino acids* and *proteins*.

Also many people with long term Chronic Depression and even Situational Depression can even be treated and even cured by these all natural brain foods found in amino acids, brain salts and proteins.

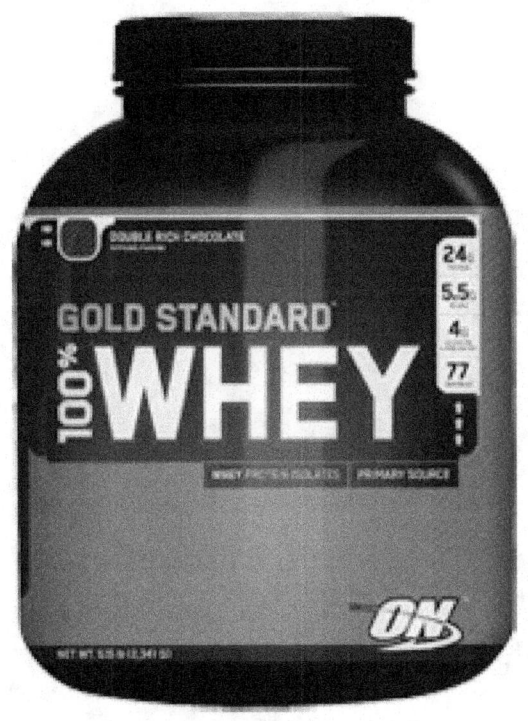

I was a perfect example of the great benefits of being healed from Chronic Depression, Situational Depression and Menopause by the simple additions of a few all natural amino acids, brain salts and proteins.

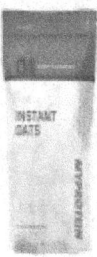

Some of which can be found naturally occurring in *eggs, almonds, pistachios* and other foods when one eats right.

That is the problem with all of our farms today. They don't think about the **consequences** they only think about the *money.*

Far too many health problems have been created by *pesticides* on our

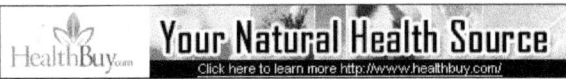

plants and trees, *hormones* and *antibiotics* fed to our livestock and poultry. **Organic** has more healthy nutrients as long as you wash it thoroughly

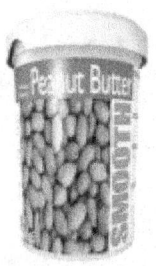

But to ensure that one is getting enough of the proteins to benefit

them than they may want to take a supplement of the <u>protein</u> itself.

Especially if they have had any kind of previous *digestive system* problems where their gut and body may not be *absorbing* the **nutrients** in their food supply.

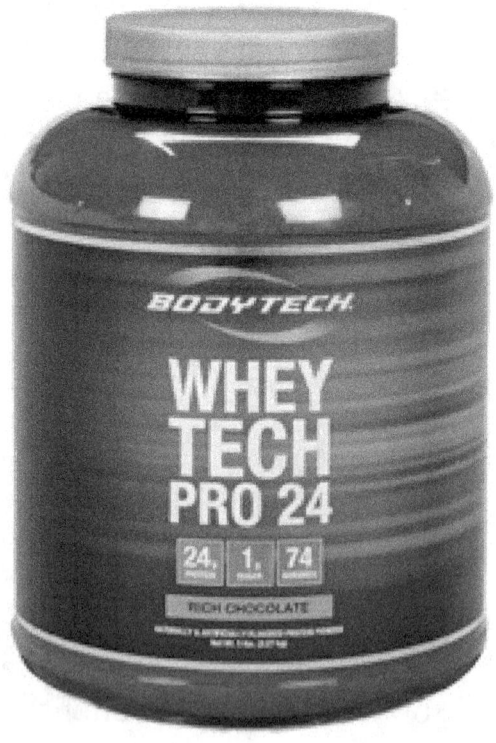

It is bad enough that our foods and even our poultry undergo so much *chemical influence* that sometimes our food can be a source for the additional health problems brought on by antibiotics, pesticides or steroids that can often times be found in our food supply.

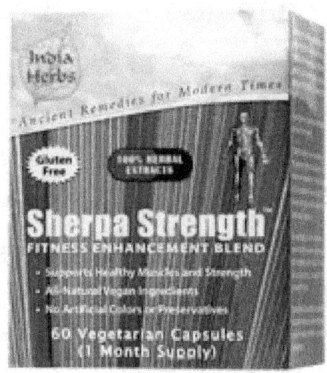

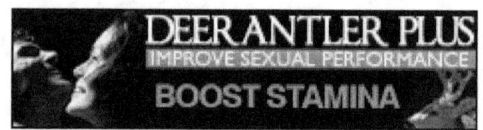

Deer Antler provides *Human Growth Hormone* which is the hormone that is most prevalent at birth and in our *youth*. As we age our body diminishes in **HGH**.

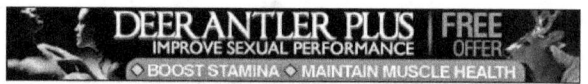

Some **Anti Aging doctors** who are considered the top specialists in the area of **Geriatrics** and Anti aging <u>highly recommend</u> Human Growth Hormone or HGH which is not readily available on the market without a prescription from a medical doctor.

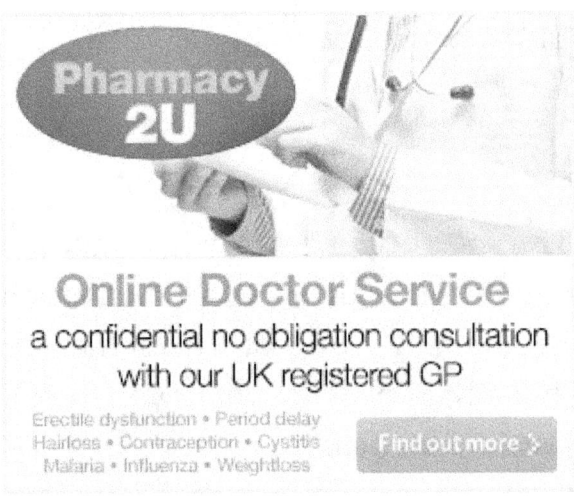
So ignore the sexual ads because
that is just an added benefit. The
greatest benefit is that it fights
depression with the <u>HGH protein</u>
and it also *turns back the clock* on
your aging.

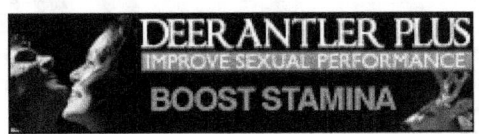

But it can be found in Deer Antler too.

The specific *proteins* that are most effective in individual products by name that you can buy from the links that I provide when you look for that particular protein are Tyrosine

 DL Phenylalanine

 Lecithin

L Carnatine

 Gaba

 Arginine

 Serine

Tryptophan.

There are other things that can be done to promote a good night sleep like taking the "Gaba" listed above at bedtime as it promotes a *healthy brain, eyes and relaxation*. It also helps fight against addictive behaviors.

Triple Magnesium is not a protein however it has been found very beneficial in overall health especially when combating women's heart health. Triple Magnesium should also be taken at bedtime because it also promotes relaxation.

Collagen is another one I take at night because it helps repair my skin and joints while it promotes rest, sleep and relaxation.

And coral calcium is not a protein either but it helps in bone and teeth health and it also helps in relaxation when taken at bedtime.

And here is an all natural sleep supplement that has Gamma amino butyric acid in it (a protein) and melatonin (which helps the brain increase in *tryptophan* in the brain which is the substance most responsible for our good mood)

You can also try Mystic Sleep an all natural sleep remedy if you need extra help until the proteins have got your hormones all the way balanced again.

They say that the most beneficial sleep for the body is if you can be sound asleep by Ten PM in your time zone and sleep for a full eight hours.

Somehow only if you are sound asleep at Ten PM is when your bodies natural antibodies kick in the most and heal your body while you are sleeping.

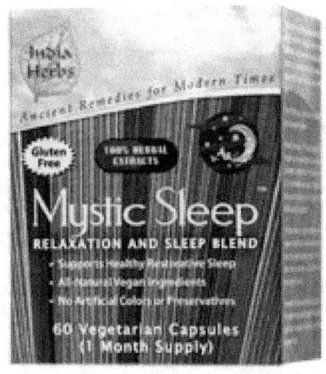

And you can also try **Berry Sleep** that is guaranteed to work.

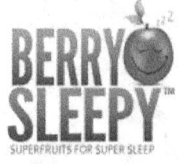

The proteins likely will cure most depressions along with many other health problems that may have been caused from hormonal imbalances or just from poor diet and lack of proteins.

You will begin to have more energy than you've had in a long time and you will begin to feel like your old self.   You will become stronger and healthier all around.

Your brain function will be quicker, sharper and clearer than before and if you had memory problems they will also begin to dissipate.

If you do not see the immediate results that I did in 2009 when I first learned of this information than it is likely that you suffer from a *different type* of **depression** than I did or you have some other health condition all together.

At which time you may need to see your own primary care physician.

There is also a great prayer line that you can always call for prayer that I use on a regular basis.

Prayers sometimes can breakthrough barriers that none other could.

I like to call *Aquilla Dove Ministries* for prayer at **1-855-200-3683** but there are many other prayer lines available too.

Like Pastor Rod Parsley of *Breakthrough Ministries* at **866-241-4292** or fill out an online prayer request here

I think it is also important that we make sure that our environments are conducive for *light and positive energy* rather than **darkness** or negative energy.

Sometimes that means one must change his environment all together.

I know when my abusive ex husband was forced by the judges court order and law enforcement to move out of my apartment so that I could move back home it wasn't long till the entire surrounding went from darkness to light somehow.

I don't know what happened but something in the spiritual changed that day.

My apartment used to be **dark, gloomy** and even dismal when he was there and I never really noticed it until he was gone.

But less than one month later I got a new eggshell colored sofa and love seat in place of my ex husbands power Lazy Boy chair that he would get drunk and pass out in time and time again.

Then I got all new colors and textures for the window coverings. I got a new coffee table that was off white and pink just like the rest of my furniture. It truly went from **darkness** to light.

My ex husband wouldn't let me have any children over to visit me nor would he even let me have anyone over to visit me.

But soon after he was gone children by the dozens started appearing out of nowhere from the neighborhood.

They wanted to come and play my piano or for me to take them to the beach. My five year youth ministry was born out of it!

The apartment went from hopeless to life, fruitfulness and joy with all the wonderful children coming to see me. We had so much fun and I would take them to church with me.

Not only did it turn their dark and dismal lives into brightness and joy of going from the ghetto apartments where we all lived and taking them to bright and wonderful church environments of fun activities for the youth and good **Christian worship songs** and wonderful people.

Environments are important! You can start by making sure that you are not letting anything negative come through your eye gates or your ear gates.

If there is anything that would bring darkness into your environment (a home, an office, or a room and even a car) than remove it immediately and ask **God** to cleanse it of any negative spirits. Ask **HIM** to *sweep* it *clean* and fill it with **HIS** *light.*

You can also speed the process by changing the *sounds* that are reverberated in the environment that you are in.

Praise and worship music are the fastest way to cleanse any darkness out of an area.

Some people prefer music **without words** like I do most of the time. I love to listen to classical music or solo piano throughout the day. That way I know that no evil communication is being transmitted through the airways.

I also know that what we speak out of our *mouths* will affect our lives and our environments.

If you have had a problem with cussing or with speaking negative things out of your mouth as I have had in my past than today is the day to change that.

Ask **God** to control your tongue by **HIS** *holy spirit.* HE tells us we can have whatsoever we ask HIM if we ask according to HIS will and if we ask in the name of Jesus.

Call those prayer lines for prayer with help to speak blessings and life out of your mouth. **Prayer** always comes in handy.

If you have a habit of keeping bad company like I once did too than you will have to decide what is more important to you it will be either your friends or your **health** and your *better future*.

Sometimes it is better to be alone than to be in the presence of those who are a negative influence in *your life*.

You also must **not** be consuming *alcoholic beverages* or *recreational* *drugs* if you truly want to get well from Depression.

Alcohol and recreational drugs are *downers* and they will only drag you down as well as drag your life to a pit of darkness and hell.

If you can find a **good church** to go to many of them have *singles groups or recovery groups* that they would love to have you as a part of.

Just find one that preaches **Jesus** and **HIS** whole **Bible** and learn their schedules and find a way to start attending.

If you really don't want to part with your friends you can give them an ultimatum to come to church with you.

Let them decide if they want to come out of the dark with you but you don't have to stay in it with them.

My prayer God will heal all who read this book from the spirit of depression. The bible says that "The thief comes to steal kill and destroy and that Jesus comes to give us life and that life more abundantly" Depression is a life stealer.

My prayer also is that God will do exceedingly abundantly above all you could hope, ask or think according to the power of God that works in you.

I pray that HE will take you from being a victim and make you a victor for HIS glory and HIS name sake.

I pray that you will fulfill all the works, plans and purposes that the Lord has created for you. And I pray that Satan's works will be destroyed off of your life, your past and your future. And I pray that **HIS Glory** will be exemplified through your life.

 In Jesus name

 Amen